less
effect

Design Your Life for
Happiness & Purpose

SAMANTHA JOY

LANDON
HAIL
PRESS

COPYRIGHT © 2018, 2022 Samantha Joy

All Rights Reserved

Published by Landon Hail Press

Paperback ISBN: 978-1-959955-06-1

Hardback ISBN: 978-1-959955-07-8

To my unborn bundle of joy:

I can only pray I am able to bring the amount of happiness and purpose to your life as you have already brought to mine

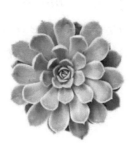

CONTENTS

SAMANTHA JOY

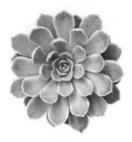

FOREWORD

WHEN SAMANTHA ASKED US to write the foreword for this book, we were very honored because we believe in her and the message that she shares within this book. Samantha is one of the rare teachers and coaches who lives her message, and it is exemplified in her everyday life. Her quality content mirrors the quality of her character.

As the owners of Maddix Publishing Company, we are able to read and publish people's books on a daily basis. On average, we read about one book per day and have developed a unique ability to identify those that offer its readers the most value.

One morning, while drinking some green tea, I started reading *The Less Effect*. I allotted an hour to review the content. However, an hour quickly passed, and I realized that I just couldn't put it down. I spent the rest of the morning partaking in the engaging stories and teachings found within this book. From the very first chapter until the last sentence, Samantha captured my attention with her transparent story and the powerful, practical content she shared.

Wow! This book has moved me deeply and caused me to evaluate some areas in my own life. *The Less Effect* lifestyle will transform your priorities and cause you to make some much-needed changes to optimize success in your life. In a world that is filled with excess, discontentment and selfishness, this book offers a timely message that is truly needed.

Not only do I spend time reading clients' books, but I've also read thousands of books on a variety of topics because I am a student of daily personal growth. I'm absolutely convinced that Samantha Joy's book must be on every bookshelf in the world. You will love this so much that you will want to buy multiple copies to give to family, friends, co-workers, and clients.

Grab a cup of coffee or tea, turn off your phone, and find a comfortable spot. Get ready to cry, laugh, and grow as a result of *The Less Effect*. Thank you, Samantha, for having the courage to write this book and share your story.

As authors of eighteen books, we know how challenging the writing process can be. You did it! Congratulations on authoring not just a book, but a tool to change the world and improve the lives of so many people in need of a breakthrough.

Matt and Caleb Maddix
Authors, speakers, and founders
Maddix Publishing

INTRODUCTION

W E'VE ALL BEEN THERE: that place where we've experienced the stress of overwhelm, when we feel like there's absolutely no way to escape it, because, well, we're too overwhelmed!

The world we live in today is specifically designed to pull our attention in a hundred and fifty different directions. It tells us what we need to know and everything we have to own in order to be our best self. Before we know it, we are caught in the endless cycle of consumerism and information overload.

Over time, we learn that once we achieve a certain status, *then* we will be successful, *then* we will be happy. It isn't long before we begin to feel inadequate, struggling to keep up with the Joneses. Our concentration and focus in our daily life becomes compromised. We put in a constant blind effort to fit the mold of who we're told we should be.

In this continuous struggle, we are left feeling lost, like we don't belong. And, as a result, we continue to feed the beast while who we are at our core and what we're meant to do on this Earth remain buried under all the madness.

The Less Effect is about becoming conscious to the areas of life that are hindering us, and clearing them out to create a life of happiness and purpose. It was born after realizing, from a very young age, I was taught more was better. This notion was subconsciously delivered to me by family, friends, the media, the educational system, and the several other channels I was exposed to throughout my life.

All I had known for the last thirty years was that to fix a problem, there was a product or person that could do it quickly and easily. This, sadly, led me down a path of major disappointment and piles of credit card debt.

It wasn't until I had my "aha moment" (a.k.a. breaking point) that I realized I was letting external factors control my destiny.

The moment I chose to become intentional with what I was allowing into my space—physically, socially, and habitually—was the moment I gained control over my life and my purpose was revealed. I was able to achieve a better sense of who I wanted to be in this world and design a life that aligned with that vision.

I discovered, by no coincidence, that having less made me much happier and massively reduced my feeling of overwhelm. Life became easier and more fulfilling. I made it my mission to declutter what was no longer serving me: less things I didn't use or love; less people who didn't add value to my life; less negative habits that held me back—all launching me into the incredible reality I have created today. The clarity and passion that can be achieved when we become the gatekeepers of our lives is an invaluable step to living the existence we've always dreamed of.

And if you don't yet know what that dream looks like, I suggest you start decluttering your own life pronto, to find out!

CHAPTER 1

The Message is in the Mess

LET'S JUST SAY I didn't have the best childhood.

I remember from a very young age—eight to be exact, realizing I was different. This may or may not have had something to do with the fact that, every day of elementary school, at 12:00 P.M. on the dot, I had to walk down to the nurse's office to take my little pink pill.

I grew up in a very dysfunctional household where physical and emotional abuse was the way to show love (or so I was led to believe). As a precautionary measure to protect against any potential past, present, or future psychological damage, pharmaceuticals became the Band-Aid. Being that I was reserved and went about my business rather than act out like a "normal" child, it was determined early on that I was "mentally ill" and required anti-depressants.

Some days, I would forget to go to take my meds, and, without fail, the school would be so kind as to page me publicly to remind me. The pointing and questions from my classmates would begin, taunting me as if I had done something horribly wrong. My olive complexion would instantly turn to a scarlet red, and I'd run out of the room, waterworks all the way to the nurse's office.

Every time this happened, it sent me a subconscious message: *"You're not good enough as you are; therefore, you need to take this pill."* It communicated to me that, in order to be "normal," I had to be chemically altered. That if I didn't deliver on who I was expected to be, the solution was to simply cover it up with something else.

As a child, this message was not entirely clear to me, but what it showed me as an adult is that everything could be solved by throwing a mask on it.

This feeling of being different and unable to measure up stuck with me for a while. If I'm being truly honest, it is something that still rears its ugly head every now and again even today, despite my major life accomplishments and praise.

What I've noticed as I've grown older (especially through working with clients in my coaching business) is how many of us are deeply affected by something from our childhood that sticks with us like a bad haircut in the eighties we could never live down. Often, it's something we've buried over the years that lives in in our subconscious, like a little green gremlin that only comes out to play the moment anything exciting happens in our lives.

It tells us all the reasons why we can't go after what we want, forcing us to resort back to our comfort zone—because, even if that's where pain lives, we know *exactly* what to expect. It holds on for dear life to the identity we've created and makes the belief that we can create a new existence seem nearly impossible.

The problem in this day and age is *we keep feeding the damn gremlin.* We acquire more things and more people to "fix" our messes. The more we pile onto our lives to cover our pain and trauma, the more he stays fed, warm, and comfy in his cushy home in our subconscious. As a result, we become clouded and overloaded, all the while losing sight of who it is we truly are and what our purpose is for being here. I quickly learned at the age of eight that to fix a problem or improve a difficult situation, I simply needed to cover it up with something else and all would be right with the world. So that is how I continued to live my life for years.

After graduating college, at the age of twenty-three, I finally decided to go off my meds. It was important to me to understand my true identity underneath it all and whether or not the drugs were crucial to my existence.

Was I actually funny? Or was that the Paxil taking over? Was I really kind and compassionate? Or was that the Zoloft making me warm in the face of others' troubles? Was I truly strong and determined? Or was that the Xanax I popped in the midst of panic? Detaching from this ritual was my first effort at a life of less without even knowing it.

And so the roller coaster began. In the absence of my chemical cocktail, anxiety came and claimed its ownership of my life. It seemed as though all the meditation and affirmations in the world were no match for the struggle I was experiencing.

Years later, things in my life came to a head. When I couldn't bear the emotional overwhelm any longer, soon after came the exit strategy. I would envision a new life, one far away from all my problems, where I could start over. Just the sheer thought of leaving it all behind put my mind at ease. And, just like that, I was gone.

I would arrive at my new home and immediately all felt right with the world. Then, months down the road, without warning, my anxiety would rear its ugly head. *But I thought I fixed this issue…*, I would reflect to myself every time. Boy, was I wrong. Every time.

It took my moving to six different cities in the course of ten years to finally realize it was time to go inward and do some soul searching. And that is exactly what I did.

The Power of Coaching

About a year ago, I was speaking with a close friend and mentor who was helping me dig deep into my personal message for my coaching business. It is important to note this man has endured struggles I would never wish on anyone, but somehow took complete ownership of his life, dug himself out of the pits of hell, and created a seven-figure business. I was in phenomenal hands.

After a bit of digging, he asked me the million-dollar question: "What is the one message you would die for?"

Well, that was a heavy one. What would I *die* for? I mean, I'm a pretty passionate broad, but there was nothing in my mind I felt *that* strongly about.

In response to my lack of response, he asked me another question: "When were the moments you felt most inspired, most alive, most in flow?"

I took a moment to look back at all the times I felt light and free to create and achieve.

I thought back on all the times I was moving around the country. It was when I escaped and arrived at my new destination that I became the most clear, the most driven, and was able to take the most action. But then it was only a matter of time before I would fall back into my old patterns and begin acquiring all the wrong things to fill the empty space.

Suddenly, it hit me like a ton of bricks: Holy shit... I was stuck in a fucking loop.

I was running away to achieve emotional relief, then, without fail, that relief would eventually disappear, and it would be time to go again. What was occurring before my exit, however, was the secret sauce: in preparation for each move, I would purge all the items in my household I didn't have any use for, I would quit jobs I had kept only for the paycheck, and I'd let go of relationships that drained me, all because I was leaving.

I had been *chasing* my happiness rather than being intentional and *creating* it.

And just like that, and my message was born:

LESS.

CHAPTER 2

A Lesson In Less

*M*INIMALISM. THE BUZZ WORD, all about owning and purchasing less things. But what does it really mean?

I stumbled upon the concept after watching the film, *Minimalism: A Documentary About the Important Things*. I discovered it shortly after having my "aha moment" and made it my mission to get my hands on anything and everything that revolved around this idea.

I already knew how exhilarated I felt after just throwing away a pile of papers, so I could only imagine the feeling that would come from implementing this on a much grander scale. Every book and blog post I read, podcast I tuned into, and expert I followed on the subject inspired me more and more into action to get rid of as many of my possessions as possible. The "KonMari" method (from Marie Kondo's book, *The Life-Changing Magic of Tidying Up*) kicked my butt into high gear, inspiring me to discard everything in my home that no longer brought me sheer and utter joy. There was no stopping me.

All of these teachings and methods helped me to finally gain control over my life. I was no longer just sitting in my mess, wishing for things to change. I was *becoming* the change by removing what did not serve me. This brought me into a newfound awareness, as if I had just walked out of Lasik eye surgery and into a whole new dimension. It quickly occurred to me that minimalism didn't have to end with my physical surroundings.

It was clear that other areas of my life desperately needed some spring-cleaning. Areas like my social environment and the places I was spending most of my time, like at work. It became apparent to me how much time I was spending around people who didn't energize me but instead completely drained me.

By disconnecting with many of these unhealthy relationships, I was further propelled to identify and clear out other negative parts of my life, like the poor habits I engaged in on a daily basis. What I discovered through this was how much we take for granted all of the freedoms we have in our lives—things like food, media, technology, and money—but how we rarely stop to think if they are being used in the most meaningful or healthy way. It became clear that many of us create addictive behaviors around these luxuries, to the point where we tend not to see it happening right in front of us. Oftentimes, we aren't even able to recognize that a problem exists. It became apparent I was no exception.

Environment Is King

The source of underlying stress and even anxiety felt by so many of us on a daily basis can be found in the unserving environments we've created for ourselves.

Often, we have grown so unaware of what we've manufactured around us that it becomes totally acceptable and even normal to most. We allow ourselves to be pulled into the status quo in order to feel comfort since questioning the current state of our lives can be a scary, arduous path. The problem is these environments we've built over the years affect us on a subconscious level, resulting in a massive energetic strain that is often unknown or undetected by our conscious mind. This happens every single day. And this is where we live and breathe. Every single day.

I'll tell you what: life becomes a lot less draining when the things around us are energetically pushing us in a healthy, uplifting direction. We suddenly find we are gaining an indescribable mental clarity in whatever we do—whether you're a public speaker presenting on stage, a professional athlete competing for the trophy, or just someone trying to find their way in the world.

The mindset piece manifests with ease, and the direction and focus of our energy become abundantly clear.

An amazing thing happens when we make the choice to scale down our lives to only what we love. Not only do we gain more control over our lives, but we are able to massively reduce stress and overwhelm. We have a much easier time making healthy decisions that reflect our best self and, as a result, uncover our greatest purpose in life.

Minimalism isn't a contest for who owns the least. It is not about scarcity.

Having less is about peeling back the layers of things and people and behaviors that do not serve us in order to discover our true self.

It is about unbecoming who we thought we *should* be in order to become the person we are *meant* to be.

It's about being unapologetically intentional with what we allow into our energy fields.

It's about having all the things we love and none of what we don't, thus creating the space for more meaningful things to enter our lives.

It's about clearing out whatever may be attached to our trauma and pain so we can rise above the limitations we've created for ourselves.

Once we do this, things becoming surprisingly simple. But I'm going to be totally honest with you: life will never be easy. Simple, yes. But easy? No.

It will *always* take work, but the work we do comes with much less mental and energetic strain when we've consciously created our life instead of letting it create us.

I want to set the record straight that more can be good, but it has to be *more of the good things*. Things that make us richer. And I don't just mean financially (although that is definitely good, and we will soon discuss why). I also mean richer in family, in experiences, in memories, in impact—all the things in life that continue to hold great meaning long after we perish. Because the truth is, at the end of the day, we all end up in a box, and we can't take our things with us.

The caveat to bringing in anything good is that most of us have an extremely difficult time identifying what that good actually looks like. That is, until we first make it a point to clear out the bad. But this experience teaches us how incredible we can feel just by choosing to no longer allow what makes us feel crappy.

It is here where the piece of intention is so crucial in our journey of minimalism. It really all just boils down to clearing out the bullshit and being purposeful with what's around us. When things start to come in, we need to become hyper-aware and say "no," if it's not going to serve us. We need to remain adamant about what we allow into our space and the choices we make for the future.

Otherwise, we are just along for the ride, adding no input along the way. Then we suddenly wake up one day and question, "How the hell did I get here?" Well, now ya' know. It's the little, tiny things every day that can completely throw us off course—*or*—catapult us in the direction of our dreams

Minimalism isn't just about discarding, but about becoming intentional about where you want to be in your life, who you want to be around, and what you want to create.

We will never have the opportunity to live out our wildest dreams until we convince ourselves it is a real possibility and we are worthy of that life. We accomplish this by surrounding ourselves with nothing but the best that uplifts and energizes us, *not* by hanging onto stuff that holds us back and perpetuates our limiting beliefs. It's when we make the conscious decision to free our environments of the dead weight around us that we are able to gain a clear depiction of who we are and what truly matters to us in our pursuit of happiness.

In an effort to help others live a more meaningful life, I've created a framework, *The Less Effect,* where I work with people to help them create that intentional environment. Every day, whether we realize it or not, we are walking through a push and pull in our day-today lives. Often, we are completely unconscious of the effect that energy has on us, yet we constantly wonder why we are not where we'd like to be.

My work is focused on helping people become more conscious of their surroundings, so they can tap into their authentic self and, as a result, design their happiest and most purposeful life.

The "M" Word

I'm going to call out the minimalism elephant in the room: *Money.* I believe this is an extremely important topic to address, since my purpose for creating *The Less Effect* was to help others design a joyful and purposeful existence, including the financial freedom to enjoy all of the wonderful things life has to offer.

I've noticed quite often how there seems to be a common misconception around the relationship between living a life of less and affluence. That if we own less and purchase less, it is acceptable to be making less, all in an effort to avoid social deception.

I find, regardless of how one chooses to live, simplistic in nature or not, money is undoubtedly a hot-button issue for many. When I adopted this new lifestyle, I, too, found myself at a crossroads around how I should address the concept of money.

* Is money good?
* Is money bad?
* Is having a lot of it contradictory to my belief system?
* Am I a fraud for wanting more of it?
* What will people think?

My personal mindset around money was a work in progress for quite some time. I thought back to how I was raised. (Because that's where all our hang-ups come from, right?)

The moment my parents divorced, money immediately became scarce since we were now split between households. My broken-home-raised readers will understand what I'm talking about. We were often told—you know that popular saying—"Money doesn't grow on trees, kids!"

For as long as I can remember, we were taught, in order to get it, you had to work really, really hard at something, doing work you may or may not enjoy. My father built his entire career on blood, sweat, and tears, running a dental practice, only to count down the days until retirement when he could start living his life. I barely saw him growing up, but in return he made a good living. That's just how it was in that generation for a lot of families.

Other common iterations of less-than-favorable money mindsets include: "Money is the root of all evil." That money is a status symbol, to show off how much a person possesses. That it's power. Many of us are led to believe money is ostentatious and opulent. When you are a person trying to live with less, it's easy to see how a negative connotation might be formed here. Well, it's time to fix that.

If you're any bit "woo-woo" like me (shout-out to my Moms), you'll understand the role of mindset in bringing in whatever it is we want into our lives. This includes our feeling around money, which most of us want more of—and that is *totally* okay. Just because we strive to streamline our lives for less doesn't mean we should subject ourselves to a life of poverty and struggle.

The notion of feeling warm and fuzzy around money instead of feeling shame or ickiness hails all the way back to 1910 and the trusty teachings of Wallace Wattles:

"There is nothing wrong in wanting to get rich. The desire for riches is really the desire for a richer, fuller, and more abundant life. And that desire is praiseworthy."

—The Science of Getting Rich

Now, if you live a minimalist lifestyle, this may be completely against everything you believe in—or even perhaps everything you've been taught to believe in. But I challenge you to open your mind to the possibility that you can—and should, in fact—possess wealth while simultaneously living a life of less. After all, minimalism is about creating the most fulfilling life possible.

I strongly believe (and have experienced with my own life, as well as with my clients') that abundance and simplicity go hand-in-hand, that you simply cannot have one without the other. Being a minimalist and having financial abundance are *not* mutually exclusive.

As a matter of fact, bringing in more money may be unavoidable after decluttering your life. The reason? You're getting closer and closer to your authentic self, and where we tend to attract the most wealth is through our true passion!

It's important to note that having a negative relationship with money is extremely prevalent. You may be thinking to yourself, "What?? I *love* money!"

Then let me ask you:

- ✓ Are you making less than you'd like to make?
- ✓ Have you plateaued at a level of income?
- ✓ Do you feel that large sums can be easily made by others but not you?

If you answered yes to any of those questions, then, subconsciously, you are hanging onto a negative relationship with money, perhaps due to a negative relationship with yourself.

I have witnessed the concept of minimalism being taken a bit too far in some cases, leading some to perceive it as not just *having* but also *making* the bare minimum.

I want to make something abundantly (pun intended) clear:

In **no** way is it acceptable to limit your own potential, financially or otherwise.

I'm guessing I've probably just rubbed a few people the wrong way who thought they were reading a book about living on virtually nothing. Sorry to disappoint, but at the end of the day, we need money to live and, even more, to thrive, and even more than that to socially impact the world (if that's a goal of yours).

The world needs you and the magical gifts only you can bring to it, which, by no coincidence, is also when we tend to make the most of it. Money is a beautiful thing when put in the right hands and used for good.

Declutter It and They Will Come

Prior to embarking on my life of less, I was living day-to-day as spiritually as possible, fully believing this was how I could manifest whatever I wanted—including money.

One day, I was listening to a podcast episode starring money-mindset coach Denise Duffield Thomas. This particular coach, bless her crass and witty little soul, touched on an absolutely critical component that was completely absent from my daily practice. You see, I was spending day after day lighting my money candle, taking deep breaths in ("I love money *ohmmmmm...*"), and out ("...and it loves me *ohmmmmm*"), rubbing my yellow citrine I'd bought for $120 on a road trip in Santa Fe with all my might... but nothing. How could I not be manifesting money when I'd chanted this to myself every day for the last ninety days? I thought this was how it's supposed to work...!?

It was the next thing she said that changed how I look at the Law of Attraction forever: "You can do all the manifestation rituals you want, but the fact is, if you don't create the space for the money to come in, there won't be anywhere for it to live." (She also compared this to rolling a turd in glitter, which is really the line that caught me, if I'm being honest).

Mind freakin' blown.

This is where I was tripping up all along. I was wishing for something to come in but had not properly prepared space for it to enter. So I started to look around me with an entirely new lens. There was *a lot* of crap cluttering my life with literally nowhere for money to come and chill with me.

Me: *Hey, Money! Make yourself comfortable and sit on top of this here box of crap I never opened in my last three moves, will ya?*

Money: *Nah, I think I'll pass and go hang at Denise's Zen garden and do some Tai Chi, instead.*

Soon after, I realized an even more critical piece of why many of the other things outside of money were missing in my life; things like a romantic partner, meaningful friendships, a fulfilling career, exciting adventures, undeniable happiness...:

There was no *room* for it, with all the junk I was holding onto.

Eureka! The code was cracked. After making it a point to massively declutter all areas of my life, I created the space to bring in thirty percent more income from my coaching business only three short months later. On top of this, I attracted better clients who were ready to step up; highly sought-after mentors who offered a massive value at the drop of a hat; and abundance in the form of humbling career opportunities and memorable life experiences—all things that had been missing from my prior life, just because I had allowed the wrong things to pile up in my energy field. Pure magic.

The truth is it is virtually impossible to bring all the yummy, good stuff into our lives when our physical, mental, and emotional states are cluttered with nonsense. By filling our space with things we don't absolutely love, we are sending an unspoken message out into the Universe that we are content with what we have and to please not surprise us with anything wonderful.

The good news? You have *all* the power to design your life exactly the way you want it. It all starts with the decision to become conscious and intentional with what you allow around you.

CHAPTER 3

Wherever You Go, There You Are

M Y PASSION FOR COACHING didn't come out of nowhere. I had always been interested in personal development for as long as I can remember.

My parents divorced when I was in second grade, and soon after, I started to notice my mother diving headfirst into self-help books. One of the first books I remember seeing on her shelf was one by Tony Robbins, *Awaken the Giant Within*. It wasn't long until Wayne Dyer, Eckhart Tolle, and Louise Hay joined the party.

I would steal these books without telling my mother because God forbid she knew I agreed with her on something! Before I knew it, I had my own personal library at my fingertips, unlocking ways to tap into my inner self and harness my greatest potential. That was the goal, anyway.

These books quickly became a security blanket through my adolescence and teenage years. I found it so fascinating that there were actual ways of training your mind to accomplish your goals. I felt like I had this competitive edge over others, because I now possessed the secret weapon of *mindset.* Speaking of "secret," it was when *The Secret*, the movie, came out (thanks for sharing, Oprah!) that my world was blown wide open. Not only did I have this ability to break through mental barriers holding me back, but I now it appeared I had the power to attract the things I'd always dreamed of. I practiced connecting my desires with feelings and made this ritual a life practice.

When I chose the pharma-free path after college, it became apparent that everything I had been studying up until this point—personal development-related, not the hundreds of thousands spent on schooling, sadly—was preparing me for the challenging road ahead. Meditation and journaling became a staple. Exercise and moving my body were a non-negotiable. I even found amateur bodybuilding in my late twenties—talk about having a strong mindset! (You try eating cold tilapia and asparagus from a Tupperware container thirty times a week...)

It was my number-one mission to master my body and mind in order to prove to myself I did not need drugs to live a healthy, emotionally balanced life. After my first bodybuilding competition, the floodgates opened with people wanting fitness and nutrition advice.

I was a certified personal trainer, something I'd completed after college, and, through my knowledge and experience, I proudly took on my first coaching client. This eventually led to a fun side-hustle that I made a cute little income on. But while I enjoyed helping people reach their potential on a physical level, there always felt like something missing. It took one special client to help me discover what that something was.

For the sake of anonymity, we will call this client Karl. Karl came to me to help him prepare for his first Ironman competition. If you're unfamiliar with what this is, let me break it down for you:

- ➢ 2.4 mile swim
- ➢ 112 mile bicycle ride
- ➢ A full marathon (26.22 mile run)

In other words, this is basically a triathlon of insane, superhuman shit—*not* for the faint of heart. You can only imagine the mindset required to dedicate oneself to a challenge of this magnitude.

I was honest with Karl in that I, myself, had never completed an Ironman (because I would likely die before even making it to the race) nor had I ever coached anyone through one. But that did not stop him from working with me, which led me to do massive amounts of research on the topic, as well as interview others who had completed an Ironman to gain an understanding of their experience.

This was an entirely new ballgame for me. While getting one's body in shape certainly takes a disciplined mindset, the level of mental energy required for such a feat, on top of the physical energy, was beyond anything I had ever coached before.

My client followed the training plan I put together but then, out of nowhere, he hit a plateau. When adding to or switching up the routine didn't resolve the issue, it occurred to me we had to work a completely different angle. This is where things got interesting.

I asked him what was happening outside his training that might be affecting his performance. Through some conversation, we uncovered that he was experiencing loads of self-doubt. Yes, this race was unfamiliar territory but, for some reason, he began to feel like it might no longer be in the cards for him. As it turns out, it was Karl's *mind* that was creating his physical limitations. Can you believe it?

I continued to delve deeper to see if I could pinpoint the reason for his discouraging mindset. It was revealed that this wasn't his first attempt in an

Ironman competition. He had tried twice before but never made all the way through the training or to the actual race.

As we continued to delve into why, he expressed that he didn't have many people around him supporting this dream of his or, frankly, believing he could do it. Therefore, his mind was telling his body achieving this goal was not possible. He happened to live in an area where health was not a priority in the local culture, to say the least; in fact, the exact opposite was encouraged. *You mean fried chicken won't increase endurance?*

That was the moment I realized how critical a supportive environment, one that aligns with our goals, plays in the role of our *identity.* Whatever we are surrounded by, especially on a consistent basis, sends us subliminal messages about who we are and what we're capable of—or, in this case, *not* capable of.

Once I got a taste of teaching others the personal development secrets I had been hoarding all these years, there was no going back. I began to dive deep into the "whys" behind all of my clients' struggles, making them look beyond the macronutrient plans and training regimens.

I would ask them questions like:

- ➤ "Why do you want to lose weight?"
- ➤ "Why has this always been a struggle for you?"
- ➤ "Why can't you accept your body the way it is?"
- ➤ "Why do you think you're not good enough?"

I wouldn't stop until we reached a breakthrough. (This made for some uncomfortable moments where many wondered what the hell they'd signed up for.) Suddenly, through this exercise, it became apparent that many of the solutions my clients initially sought from me were not, in fact, what they desired at all.

There was no better feeling than serving my clients on this entirely new level, helping them to break through physical, mental, and emotional plateaus. All of my years of studying self-help gurus and creating this competitive advantage for myself had opened the door for me to create the same for others and lead them to new heights they'd never thought possible.

There was nothing else I could imagine myself doing with my life.

About a year later, I slowly transitioned into mindset coaching and left the world of fitness behind me. My focus on clients moving forward was getting to the root of their limiting identities, and reverse engineering what led them to living in these identities in the present moment.

The Identity Code

The Oxford Dictionary defines the word *identity* as: *The fact of being who or what a person or thing is.*

Author Larry Ackerman takes this meaning a step further and describes *The Identity Code* as "a person's unique characteristics that determine their potential and capacity for success." In other words, a person's success is a direct correlate of their individual attributes that make up who they are. Now, let's dive into this a bit more. After all, identity is the foundation for what makes us who we are today. (Even *Oxford* says so!)

While this may be news to some of you, it may be terribly obvious to others: our identity is deeply rooted in our *stories*.

When I say stories I mean how our experiences throughout our lives have directly shaped us. From these experiences, we've created interpretations, which have later led to beliefs about ourselves. This is the story we live by. Some of our stories were written from being told we were capable of anything and destined to be a major success! But most of us were not so lucky to experience this Lifetime-movie marathon.

Some of us are able to rewrite this story, but not without drastic change that leads to a life transformation. Most of us still live by the story we created in childhood without consciously knowing it, which is not a surprise, given how our identity is indoctrinated into us.

The largest reason for continuing to live in our story is resistance to change. Our identity is further solidified through predictability, which allows us to conform and avoid risk, as well as by "self-verification," which keeps us trapped. If we change, then we can't predict what comes next, which leads to major discomfort.

Living in an old, unserving identity can come at a major cost. Just think about Mike Tyson, who squandered away his $300 million fortune and ended up in bankruptcy. His identity was rooted in debt; therefore, his pattern was to spend more than he made.

The same goes for all the lottery winner stories we hear, about a family with a household income less than $30,000 who wins $40 million and then has nothing to show for it a year later. This is commonly due to a scarcity mindset that stems from the deep-seated belief that being financially free will never be an actual possibility. At the end of the day, identity governs value, and if we're stuck in a story that says we are not worthy of what we want, that's exactly where we will end up, regardless of what opportunities come our way.

"But what does identity have to do with minimalism?" you ask. The answer is this: Everything we engage with on a daily basis—our things, our people, our jobs, our actions—is a direct reflection of our identity and the stories that continue to reinforce it.

It is absolutely crucial to become conscious of the stories we have told ourselves before we can take the steps to create massive change in our lives, including the act of discarding things we have held onto so tightly.

When we become aware of our current identity, it is likely it may not be one that is serving us to our highest potential. Therefore, a transformation is in order. That is where this all comes full circle.

How do we change our identity? The answer is simple. We change our *environment.* We strip away all that is attached to that old identity, anything that is no longer serving us to break free of whatever has been holding us back. This is single-handedly the most powerful step in rewriting our stories and allowing us to become the best versions of ourselves and live our best lives.

Our identity helps to explain where all of our stuff came from. "Stuff" can be interpreted in many ways, but in this case it is all of the things we possess, including our physical items, our relationships, our daily habits, and our general outlook on life. Everything we think, everything we say, everything we do, even everything we own is a direct reflection of the person we believe ourselves to be and the capabilities we believe ourselves to possess.

Remember how I moved six times in ten years yet continued to have anxiety? That was because I was living in an old identity, one that said I wasn't acceptable as I was, so I kept grasping for things outside myself in the hope it would make things better. Every time I decluttered and moved, it was inevitable I would go back to that old story, acquiring a bunch of crap, repeating the same behaviors that aligned with that identity.

When I made it a point to consciously change my world around me and become diligent in my pursuit of my true identity, that is when I was able to step into my greatest potential and begin living my most meaningful life.

And so can you.

CHAPTER 4

Like Attracts Like

*I*N MY FIRST YEAR of mindset coaching, I created what appeared to be a large impact in others' lives, yet I was experiencing challenges in my own life, despite applying all the principles I taught my clients.

The work I was doing was extremely fulfilling, however, I still managed to struggle with bouts of anxiety. I casually chalked this up to it just being a biological part of who I was, without giving much thought to the possibility that it could ever be any different. Isn't that what we all do? Sweep our junk under the rug because heaven forbid we actually face the reality that we can change it?

This, of course, was prior to embarking on my epic journey of minimalism. At the time, I was still working at a job that didn't align with my passion, nor did I feel the slightest bit valued at the company. This wasn't some super-big secret, buried and unknown to me. I was *fully* aware of my sheer hatred for 99.9% of the things that were demanded of me. I punched in, putting all my joy on hold until I punched out, and only then was it time to partake in any fulfilling activities. But that was acceptable because I was making a decent living, at least by my own limited standards at the time.

I lived in a beautiful apartment I paid way too much for that was covered in a surplus of things, casually scattered about with virtually no method to the madness. I had packed boxes that sat there for months as decoration, constantly telling whoever I had over, "Don't mind those—I just recently moved here," as the days continued to pass me by and the boxes continued to collect dust.

It was possible many of these boxes contained knitting needles from my hipster days on the NYC subway or my iPhone 3 with a hairline crack in the screen, making it totally worth saving (wouldn't you?)—none of which I was too thrilled to own, given they had remained packed throughout my last three moves. The remaining things were pretty much whatever I'd grabbed when exiting the last apartment I'd shared with my ex: a.k.a. cursed merchandise.

I created friendships with questionable people out of necessity, since the alternative meant being alone, which would *obviously* be so much worse. This meant a lot of nights out at the bars downtown, attempting to blend in with the unfamiliar territory of way too much alcohol and way too little sleep for what my body was used to.

Don't get me wrong: I'm pretty sure Abba named their hit song "Dancing Queen" after me. But waking up at 11 A.M. the next day, only to scarf down a large pizza in my polka-dot pj's and pass out five hours later, was too reminiscent of my college days. And not in the good way like when you attend an alumni game and sing fight songs with your old buddies you haven't seen in ten years.

Complementing my meditations and journaling, I binge-watched Netflix to escape the confusion and dissatisfaction of my current situation. I'd be sure to get my daily quota of Facebook scrolling at least ten times a day. I mean how else would I know what's going on in the world?

Television and social media were not the only things I was binging. My former bodybuilding days left me with a bit of a body dysmorphia hang-up, which often resulted in my overindulging in food. I knew better than to have anything unhealthy in my house. I was a health nut, or so everyone knew me as. This was certainly outwardly true, but, every now and then (more times than I'd like to admit), I would give in to that little demon inside of me whose main goal in life was my self-sabotage.

Now, for those of you reading this, you can clearly spot the obvious sources of my anxiety. What I was experiencing on a daily basis was certainly not ideal, that's for damn sure. But what I failed to notice at that point was not that I was *experiencing* those hurdles; it was that I was unconsciously **creating** them.

Let that one sink in for a moment.

It was my lack of awareness of what I owned and who I engaged with that led me to this place, year after year after year. This realization threw me for a major loop, given all the constant personal development work I had done for so many years.

This oblivion is not uncommon. In fact, it is the *most* common thing I see with my clients and, to be frank, in most people I cross paths with.

After experiencing what it was like to become hyper-aware of my surroundings and remain diligent in removing what didn't belong, I knew this was something people desperately needed. When I began applying *The Less Effect* to others' lives, it became clear just how insidious this epidemic truly was.

Many of us have an extremely difficult time identifying these red flags when it comes to our own lives. We fail to examine what we've acquired and created throughout the years—physically, socially, and habitually. Before we know it, we're living an existence that ranges anywhere from monotony to overwhelm to complete misery. Sometimes it gets so out of control that we wake up feeling like imposters in our own lives. It isn't until we become conscious to our choices in these areas that we are able to escape the crap trap.

We Are Energy, Energy Is Us

Something extremely important to learn early in life, if you haven't already is this:

We are Energetic Beings.

Whether you believe in Jesus, Allah, the Unicorn Queen of Saturn, or your pet rock, Marvin, there is no denying we humans absorb the energy of our surroundings. Now, this can be taken several ways:

We can look at it objectively, in that the entire physical Universe is made up of pure energy and vibration. For example, light is a form of vibration. The electromagnetic wave spectrum of light produces colors, which are simply wavelengths that vibrate at various frequencies. As we know, colors are found in the many things we own in our home, on our bodies, at our offices, in public spaces, etc. It's why they say brighter colors like yellows are good for the kitchen, to keep us awake, while warmer colors like beige are better for the bedroom, to put us to sleep.

Another common vibration we experience every day? Sound. Slow, bassy music has a lower vibration, and faster, energetic music has—you guessed it—a higher vibration. This is the reason we tend to feel down during a melancholy ballad versus feeling upbeat when we hear a peppier tune. Sounds also come from people's mouths (fortunately or unfortunately) that can make us feel like we're ready to rock or ready to go home and take a nap.

Another way to approach the concept of energy is in the more metaphysical sense, based on our emotions and spiritual belief system. Simply put, we feel happier and more energized when we're in a space that we love, around people we love, doing things that we love. We can feel a major drop in our energy levels when find ourselves in situations that do not align with our core values or meet our needs.

Why is it we feel so uplifted when we're on vacation and so drained when we're at work? Why do we feel like anything is possible after attending a motivational seminar but discouraged about life after hanging around our mindless "friends" at the bar?

It's simple. We are attracted and energized by the things that portray our highest self and depleted by everything else. To sweeten the pot, when we are on that higher wavelength, we tend to attract more good things. The vibration of our bodies on both a physical and non-physical level has been shown to have a noteworthy effect on our capacity to attract positivity. As our vibration increases, the stronger our pull becomes to bring in whatever thoughts we create in our mind.

Whether you are a follower of science or your heart, there is no denying what we surround ourselves with has a massive impact on our emotional and energetic state. This goes for the items in our household we've collected over time, the relationships we've held onto year after year, our jobs we've remained loyal employees at, and the habits we've formed, including the way we speak to and treat ourselves on a daily basis.

Case in point? Everything around us, every second of every day matters! It's what brought us to where we are in this very moment in time and what will continue to move us on the exact same path until we make the conscious decision to be more protective with our precious energy.

CHAPTER 5

Home is Where the Organized Joy Is

*T*HERE'S NO ARGUMENT that decluttering our home, or even a small area of our home like a closet, for example, leaves us feeling refreshed and renewed. It's as if we suddenly sprout a cape and can take on the world.

If that's the case, then the question remains: why do we continue to have so much stuff? It seems logical we would feel better with fewer things crowding us, yet we somehow find ourselves among a mountain of objects we don't even use or, in worse cases, don't even remember we have. The *LA Times* discovered that the average American household owns 300,000 items. Who has enough time or energy to deal with that much crap? I sure don't. And I'm going to guess you don't either.

What's ironic about how we treat our spaces is that we as humans are actually recognized as having an intrinsic awareness of our environment and we seek out surroundings that possess pleasing characteristics to us. Yet, when it comes to our own homes, many of us tend to miss the mark.

You may be thinking to yourself that you love the space you've created, but is everything in your space something you can say truly enriches your life? If the answer is no, then it is likely you're experiencing some degree of energetic strain. Our environments have the ability to create or reduce stress; keeping things around us that do not add value to our lives—whether in plain sight or not—creates stressors.

That novelty Betty Boop figurine you got from your aunt's trip to Vegas that's sitting in the corner of your desk? Energetic strain. *No offense, girl—you're totally adorbs—but you do absolutely nothing to enrich my life.* Same goes for the bowling ball you haven't pulled out in ten years hiding in the back of your closet. Let's get real: that thing is now a certified paperweight.

When we are under stress, we are not in a state that allows us to create, to take action, or to attract positivity into our space. Instead, we experience feelings of overwhelm and mental fogginess.

It's like when I had my breakthrough. I was the most productive and the most at ease when I had the least cluttering me. This is still absolutely true to this day for me and must constantly be kept in check. Hell, it took me a round of decluttering and organizing to be able to write anything worth reading in this book!

Also, think of how much time we've spent in our lives looking for things. Imagine if we didn't have as many things to look for—that's time not only saved looking in the first place, but also less time spent looking for the things we still own, because we would know exactly where they are!

The point I'm emphasizing here is what clutters the home clutters the mind, even the items out of our line of sight. And if you think these items we stash away have "no effect" on us, given that we do not pay them much attention, you're sorely mistaken. This is precious real estate that could otherwise be organized and simplified, recreating that same calming effect within our bodies and minds. Every square inch matters.

The Consumerism Trap

Many of us look for quick fixes to fill a void, one that is likely to stay empty the more we try to fill it with stuff.

Consumerism is a never-ending cycle. It's a trap that lures us in by making us believe solutions can be found in inanimate objects. The problem is we are only treating the symptom—temporarily at that. Until we make the decision to peel away the layers of junk to reveal the root cause of what is ailing us, we will forever be stuck in the feeling that we never have enough.

Hallmark holidays are the crown jewels of consumerism. It's like when consumerism had their marketing meeting, this idea was at the top of the whiteboard.

Listen, I don't blame people for having expectations regarding the socially accepted traditions and rituals around holidays; they have been indoctrinated in us throughout our entire lives. But it's important that we recognize, as we grow into adults, what is truly important at the end of the day.

Let me ask you: when you gather for a holiday, what do you remember ten years later? Probably when your Uncle Louie shot beer out of his nose, laughing at your joke. Or holding your newborn nephew for the very first time. It's likely you won't remember a gift you unwrapped and stored in your closet months later.

I have a friend who told me he once had a girlfriend break up with him on Valentine's Day after she had been expecting something from him and he didn't deliver. He learned his lesson about the importance of communication and told his now-wife, when they started dating, not to expect anything on this day. Not now, not ever.

This may sound harsh to you ladies (or even some of you men out there), but there are a few things here that I totally admire. First off, shouldn't every day be an expression of love? Secondly, why does our expression of love have to be delivered through a physical object? And last, how much more meaningful is it when we receive that love without expectation or force, but, instead, naturally, whenever it strikes? Celebrating others in our life does not need to be scheduled to a socially accepted calendar. Furthermore, we do not need to purchase material things to prove our love, admiration, or pride in another.

Often, our choices, our habits, and our surroundings seem completely acceptable to most of us. I see this all the time. What may seem totally normal to us, another person would look at and run straight for the hills.

How do we get into this mess in the first place (literally)? The truth is the majority of people look for extraneous solutions to their problems, oftentimes completely unaware they are doing so. I certainly was guilty of this.

What happens with this external seeking is it becomes a learned behavior and eventually results in a disconnected self. What I mean by this is, when we continue to answer the calls outside ourselves, over time we become a slave to the demands of what others want and whatever is expected of us without much question. These demands come from various places, including people closest to us, co-workers, school teachers, acquaintances, and society. Eventually, we go on autopilot, and our impulses are driven by this disconnected self. It is here that consumerism cashes in big time. It preys on those who feel like there might be something missing in their life, convincing them the solution can be found in having more.

A majority of people fall victim of this, and it's no coincidence, given we live in a world handcrafted to perfect the art of consumerism and overwhelm. There are a million and one channels communicating with us at all times that we willingly (subconsciously or not) invite into our energy field. We absorb subtle and sometimes not-so-subtle messages through these channels every day that constantly instruct us of what we need. They're essentially telling us we are not acceptable as we are and, in order to be "better," we need to have more, do more, be more... More, more, more.

Marketing makes this a tough trap to escape. It's planted in our television shows, our news, our social media, our apps, and our drives to work. If we want to properly fit into society, it is important we own the latest and greatest everything, or so we are brainwashed to think. Yes, you are brainwashed.

Some of us are not able to afford these luxuries, which creates a feeling of unworthiness. The mission of consumerism is to confuse a person's "want" with "need," resulting in a non-negotiable purchase. This has led many people into handsome debt, which often makes them feel cornered in a job where they are unfulfilled, for fear they will not be able to support themselves otherwise. I know. I was one of those people.

Before we know it, we are living amongst piles of things we don't wear, don't use, don't feel any joy from, but keep around for some crazy reason. We dedicate spaces of our house to storing these items, many of which we neglect to acknowledge for months, sometimes years. Other times, we pay money for square footage at an offsite location to hold these things while we pay for their rent. I mean how insane is that when you really think about it? We're essentially renting items we've already paid for in full, and we're not even using them!

So why would we engage in such ludicrous behavior? Why would we consciously keep pouring money into items we own? Or even why would we hang onto these items in the first place, if they're not adding value to our lives?

There are several explanations for why we find ourselves holding on for dear life to things we don't necessarily really enjoy. One reason is explained by the concept of *sunk cost bias*. It relates to our tendency to continue investing in an unfavorable outcome because of the original investment we've already made in it. We keep the item and sometimes even force use of it, so we don't feel like we've actually lost it, regardless of the fact that there is little to no fulfillment from it.

This is not a huge surprise, as humans are extremely loss averse. Sometimes the continuous investment isn't money at all, but time or energy. This is especially true with material items we own. Ladies, did you ever continue wearing a pair of pumps that cut your feet like glass just because of the price tag? Yeah, ya did.

As crazy as this sounds, we are all guilty of it because, in the end, we all want to avoid suffering a loss, especially if it's a pricey one. To have to admit to making a foolish purchase in our minds looks much worse than enduring the pain (physical and emotional) to save face. It's important to make the logical decision of quitting while you're ahead because, the fact is, the more money, time, and energy we spend investing in something that doesn't fulfill us, the less we can spend investing in something that does.

Another compelling concept that analyzes our need to hang onto material things is explained by the *endowment effect*. This involves placing a higher value on something we already own than on something we do not. Various studies have been conducted to explore this concept. However, in the classic study that has received the most attention, participants were asked to assess the value of coffee mugs to prove this theory.

Two groups were asked to sit in separate rooms. The first group was given mugs and told they now owned the mugs. The second group was simply shown the mugs and was able to inspect them visually. Individuals in both groups were asked to report their perceived value of the mugs. The individuals in the group who owned their mugs consistently valued them higher than the individuals who only inspected them, and in some cases said they would prefer to keep their mugs rather than sell them. This showed the rapid pace at which attachments are formed with an item after ownership is established.

Sometimes, our resistance to letting go simply comes down to waste. The item could be one of very little value, but perhaps we grew up with not very much. The minute we even come close to thinking about discarding something, a hologram of our mother pops out of the woodwork to scold us, and we immediately feel immense guilt.

When we're given gifts, we often feel obligated to hang onto them for fear of insulting the gifter. This also goes for cards in the mail, as well as wedding and baby announcements.

Other times, we live in the "just in case" scenario. This is my favorite. Better keep all that boating equipment collecting dust in the basement from that boat we sold twenty years ago... Ya' know, just in case! This is on a much grander scale than the tire pump you keep for the bike you no longer own, but you get the idea.

The sad thing is, if we totaled up the square footage that stores these items, we could likely downgrade to a smaller home, and the amount saved in housing would far outweigh the cost to rent the items when needed.

A common subset of this excuse that I see quite often is pride. You know that set of golf clubs you last used ten years ago at the club with your buddies? The ones you keep *just in case* you play again one day? Well, the jig is up. We both know you're not going to play again after that back surgery you had last fall. You're keeping them because you're not ready to let go of the fact that life has changed. There is definitely some emotional pain associated with clearing out items that remind us of our glory days, but, believe it or not, it's the actual act of holding on to them that perpetuates that pain as a reminder.

We hold on to items that are sentimental to us as mementos. I believe these are the most challenging things to let go of. Sometimes, it's a keepsake to commemorate an important life event, something to refer back to when we want to experience it again.

Let's be real for a moment. How many times does this *actually* happen? That we actually go back through our memory boxes in detail and relive an experience? Pretty much never. They stay tucked away in a closet, regardless of the sentiment they may hold.

In other cases, these keepsakes are the way we remember loved ones whom we have lost. We feel, by letting go of the physical item, we are letting go of the person. This is where discarding becomes extremely difficult. The important thing to remember here is that memories are eternal. We hold them in our hearts, so, no matter what physical item is removed, we will always have that person with us.

There are times when we may not even be aware that a lot of what we own has got to go. The reason being? They are a representation of our story, the one we tell ourselves that holds us back from our most amazing life. Likely it's a story linked to an old identity that we no longer wish to entertain.

At the end of the day, whatever we've created around us is a direct reflection of how we view ourselves. If we have items that are tattered, falling apart, unusable, or outdated, then we do not think very highly of ourselves and do not believe we are worthy of attracting anything better into our life. This has a ripple effect into the Universe to send us more crap that aligns with that story. If we want to shed an old identity that no longer serves us, there is no better way than by letting go of items attached to that old identity.

The constant battle so many of us are fighting is that we become so attached to our things that it becomes questionable whether we own our possessions or our possessions own us. When we put such a large focus on material things, they become a priority in our life: the source of our daily conversations, our arguments, even competition and bragging. This focus subconsciously convinces us that our property is a part of us.

Well, I'm here to give you a big ol' reality check:

We are NOT our things.

Yes, our environment is a reflection of our self-worth, but what it contains does not determine who we *are*. We create such huge attachments to our things that we completely forget what is truly important in life.

If our houses burned down today, would we suddenly become half a person? No. We would thank God for our survival and likely reprioritize how we view things.

I've known people who have suffered this calamity, and their outlook on life is extremely refreshing, to say the least. Hopefully, this is not something you have to go through, in order to realize this truth.

The sooner we recognize what really matters, the sooner we can break free of the consumerism trap and unveil the truest version of ourselves so we can embark on a life of fulfillment and joy. It's out there waiting for you. You just need to polish off all the gunk to see it!

CHAPTER 6

You Are What You... Hang Out With

I LOVE TO THINK about our social environment using the "Coffee Shop Theory." (I just made that up, but stay with me here.)

Think of the last time you were at [insert local coffee shop here], and you were waiting in line. We've all witnessed the irritable grump who can't get through the line fast enough, complaining the whole way to the counter about the shitty service. But every now and then there's someone who turns around, flashes us a big smile, and asks us how our day is going.

Who would you rather share your skinny vanilla latte with? I personally prefer option B. It's the simple act of putting out a positive vibe that invites other positive people in. People are not attracted to misery... unless, of course, they are miserable people. The more you hold yourself back by hanging around with people who do not motivate and inspire you, the more you will continue to attract those same people into your life.

When I decided to take minimalism a step further, I knew that, just like my physical environment, my social environment needed some serious decluttering. I believe many of us collect people throughout our life journey, much like we do material objects. We usually fail to take periodic inventory of what we have accumulated... or, in this case, "who."

Whether we want to take responsibility for it or not, the people we choose to surround ourselves with have a massive impact on where we are today. This not only includes our closest friends, but our family members, our co-workers, those we see at church, our neighbors, parents at the PTA meetings, and other miscellaneous people we come into contact with.

You've likely heard the Jim Rohn quote: "You are the average of the five people you spend the most time with." I've always been fond of this quote, because I appreciate the intended message: who we spend the most time with has an influence on who we are, as people. There is no denying that.

Well, I like to take this idea a step further and say: "You are the sum of *all* the people you spend *any* time with." And why do I say this? You guessed it: *energy.*

We put out and receive energy every single day, and we are influenced by others' presence, whether we ask for it or not. While we certainly absorb the most energy from the people we spend the most time with, we are also affected by others we come into contact with throughout our day, regardless of intimacy level. And our interactions create a domino effect, where one reaction can affect another, affecting another, and so forth. This can change the entire outcome of our day.

I apologize to the diehard stoics in the house who claim they are immune to this stimulus, but for the rest of us—just think back to the last time you spent the day at the DMV and tell me how motivated you felt to take on the world after you left. Moral of the story: it's critical we limit ourselves to as little negativity and fewest stressful situations as possible.

Our actions each day are driven by stimuli that either energize or drain us. A lot of this will sound familiar to the effects we experience with our physical environment, but our social environment has an especially large impact on well-being each day.

As humans of the Earth, we are subjected daily to an energetic exchange. When we are encouraged, we feel lifted up and limitless. When we are discouraged, we feel depleted and powerless. This alone is the reason our circle is so paramount to our success. Do you think Bill Gates chose to hang around with a bunch of haters in his spare time while he was building Microsoft? I'm going to go out on a limb and say he did not.

The effect of other people's energy on us is, I believe, best demonstrated through a study conducted at Bielefeld University in Germany, where researchers confined multiple plants to a space, testing their ability to derive secondary energy sources for growth. The team of researchers cut off the typical sources of energy that promote photosynthesis, which caused the plants to pull energies from the other plants. This was accomplished by the plants creating enzymes that digested the cellulose from the other plants in order to grow.

The outcome provided potential evidence that people can absorb energy from one another in a similar fashion. The researchers compared the human organism to a plant in that it draws necessary energy to feed certain emotional states, in addition to other vital energies like food, water, and sunlight. This can result in either energizing cells or catabolizing cells, depending on the emotional catalyst.

I find this study fascinating because it breaks down the actual science behind an organism's ability to absorb surrounding energies, along with the positive as well as harmful effects that can occur, as a result. So many of us go through life never questioning the relationships we've formed and how they have played a role in forming us, for better or worse.

Some of our closest friends are the ones who drain us, but we have history, so we keep them around. Sometimes we have family members who hold us back, but they are blood, so we learn to deal with them. Other times it's our coworkers or our boss cutting us down, but that is how we feed ourselves, so we force ourselves to tolerate their poor treatment. We condone these behaviors and allow these vampires to continue sucking the life out of us, unaware of their extremely detrimental effects. *No bueno*.

The More You Know

Unhealthy relationships can come in many forms. They can be outright toxic cases where we are able to easily identify the negative repercussions. But others can be difficult to detect.

How do we recognize them? Luckily (or perhaps not so luckily), I've had some experience with these types in my day. The biggest weapon we have in avoiding their harmful ways is by understanding the various breeds we encounter.

One I am always sure to steer clear of personally is the *downer*. We've all had one of those. This is the person who, no matter what the circumstance, is wired to look at the glass as half empty. By now, I can only hope all of you readers understand the importance of positivity in attracting positive things. This person is essentially offering you shotgun on their road trip to misery.

Another type we often come into contact with is the *complainer*. They are a remix of the downers but much more vocal in their message that life sucks a big one and will explain every single way in which their happiness is being intercepted. No, thank you.

Many of us have struggled with the *victim* or *martyr,* who finds fulfillment in soliciting guilt. These people believe that everything happens *to* them and any negative outcome they experience is the cause of another person. They simply cannot get out of their own way, and they do nothing to encourage or support our successes. We tend to hang onto these people more tightly because of the sympathy we feel for them due to their low self-esteem. Ironically, our sticking around only encourages their masochistic behavior.

What about the *melodramatics*? Now, those are a good time! Not. These types jump at the chance to make a mountain out of a molehill. They are experts at creating problems to drum up excitement, are fueled by conflict, and thrive from taking you along for the ride.

Have you ever dealt with someone who always puts themselves first? Then you've got a *narcissist* on your hands. Their main goal in life is for others to feed their ego. Their often warm and charming ways are a strategic move to gain your trust, which they will later use for their own personal agenda.

An extension of the narcissist is the *selfish* types, who will take whatever you give them with no reciprocation. Over time, we may create a learned behavior around this kind, setting a subconscious standard around the dynamic of the relationship that you owe them. Perhaps you believe your acts of service, selflessly expecting nothing in return, are a reflection of being a quality friend. Unfortunately, this is not the case, as all healthy relationships should be mutually beneficial.

Toxic relationships, while they are often the most obvious to spot, can be the most challenging to break away from. Despite the pain they may be causing, we are receiving some level of payoff that may be driven by an old identity, much like our attachments to our things. (You will continue to hear me say this throughout the book, as it is such an important component of designing a more fulfilling life.) We may believe that we don't deserve better. We may be codependent. We may fear being alone. Whatever the reason is, there is no case in which surrounding ourselves with harmful people is good for us. Period.

Many of us have relationships with people we feel aren't necessarily harming us but are not really helping us, either. We may talk about the weather or who won the big game last night. But these are not people who are setting the world on fire.

I'm going to share something with you that a former coach once shared with me that I wish I knew a lot earlier. If you want a better life, it's going to require massive change and major shifts in your thinking. This *cannot* be accomplished when we surround ourselves with small-minded thinkers who are incapable of encouraging our potential.

I know this may sound severe, but we only get one life, and we must treat our limited time on Earth as the precious asset it is. These idle conversations occupy valuable time we could be using to engage with others who propel us forward in the direction of our dreams. While these neutral relationships aren't doing any real, visible damage, they are like cement in the floor of our current reality and will never allow us to reach our higher self.

In the case of unhealthy relationships, this is where we often experience the *sunk cost bias* yet again. We have invested so much time and effort into a relationship that we hang onto it, praying for a different outcome. If you've tried to resolve the issues to the best of your ability, it may be time to call it quits. Staying in an arrangement that hurts both parties helps no one become better or happier people. Those are just the cold hard facts.

We can get a better idea about people who might be holding us back us by considering our most significant relationships in our life today—in business and career, friendships, romantic partnerships, family, and any others. Think about what these people are actually bringing to the table.

How do they make you feel? Be honest with yourself. It may even help to consider what you're bringing to the table, to identify a potential imbalance or lack of effort on your part that shows you are no longer invested. If you're able to determine that any of your relationships appear to be hurting you, it's important to address them. But if you're experiencing continuous abuse, it is not worth continuing the relationship, no matter how much time, money, energy, or love you've put into it.

Our social environment can dictate the trajectory of our life. While what we do inevitably falls on us, not one person who has achieved massive success or experienced immense joy in this world got there by choosing people who dragged them down. No one is worth throwing away our dreams for. Cut your losses, and get ready for some beautiful change ahead.

CHAPTER 7

We Are What We Repeatedly Do

IF YOU WANT TO LEARN about a person, watch their daily habits. Everything we do reflects the way we feel about ourselves. Just like our things and our relationships... Surprise! That's why this piece is so crucial to declutter when designing our best life.

To begin to design a life full of meaning, we must discard the habits that hold us back from our pursuit. I don't think anyone can say that they've kicked all their bad habits. I certainly can't. But what I can say is I'm a hell of a lot better than I used to be just by becoming conscious of the severe damage certain habits were causing me.

When I began mindset coaching, creating a healthy routine that supported my clients' goals was priority. As we know, it's the little things we do every day that get us closer to our goals. While initially adopting a positive routine seemed to go great, I saw a lot of my clients fall off those routines within months, weeks, and sometimes days of implementing them.

What I had failed to do was bring to light the negative habits they were engaging in and then assist them to kick those to the curb first. I had assumed (and you know what that does) that putting positive habits in place would eventually remove the negative ones naturally. Well, clearly this was not the case. Once, I began to dig deep into what behaviors were holding them back, we worked on eliminating those before adding back in healthy ones. In order to create a healthier daily routine, we had to remove the bad habits taking up time and space.

In an effort to understand where these unfavorable behaviors come from, let's first take a look at how habits are formed.

Every habit starts with a psychological pattern called a "habit loop," which consists of a three-part process. It starts with a cue or trigger that tells your brain to go into autopilot and act on that urge. Next is the routine or the action itself. This is what we think about, typically, when we call something a habit. Finally comes the reward or "payoff." This is basically the prize that trains our brain we should repeat this behavior again, thus repeating the cycle.

These behaviors are traced back to the *basal ganglia*, the part of the brain in charge of developing our memories, emotions, and pattern recognition. The *prefrontal cortex*, which you may be familiar with, is the part responsible for making decisions. What's fascinating about this section of the brain is that as soon as a behavior becomes learned, it goes into sleep mode, essentially putting the behavior on autopilot. While this is good news, since it creates mental capacity to dedicate to other things, it can be dangerous when the learned behavior is one that is sending us up shit's creek.

An interesting link has been made between our habits and our environment. Studies have actually shown that quitting smoking while on vacation reduces the probability of relapse. This is due to the fact that all your old cues and "rewards" have been removed. As a result, there is an ability to form a new pattern that is more likely to be sustained.

Other scientific research has shown that it's never too late to break a habit. The best way to change a habit is to become conscious of how it was actually formed. When we become aware of the triggers, cues, and rewards, we are forced to see how these show up in our behavior. Therefore, it becomes easier to change.

Control Your Habits, Control Your Life

There are numerous pacifying activities we choose to engage in that completely divert us from creating the new, awesome life we've always dreamed of. Let's call out a huge one that is impacting most if not every human with access to technology today: social media.

It has been reported that, in the course of one day in 2017, the average American adult spent approximately two hours and fifty-one minutes on their smartphone. It's safe to say this has become an addiction throughout society. This comes as no surprise, since we've recently learned that many apps have been specifically designed to manipulate our brain chemistry to create an addictive response. This is known as "intermittent rewards," where the app's algorithm monitors your activity and feeds you notifications periodically, which keeps the scroller on the hook.

Social media has become a hot topic nowadays, since it can be used for so much good—connecting us with like-minded communities and people, as well as growing our businesses—but it has also been traced to causing psychological damage and emotional stress. This does not come as a shock, given that advancements in technology have created a world of instant gratification while diverting us further away from human interaction. Many technologies drive us to look constantly for our next feeling of excitement or happiness within a device.

This has affected how we engage socially in a major way. Why would we choose to leave our homes to mix it up with new people when we can order a pizza—and really anything else we could ever want—from the comfort of our 500-thread-count Egyptian cotton sheets? And that rush we feel when receiving likes, comments, and messages? That's dopamine, my friends. Yes, the same dopamine that is generated from activities like working out, laughing with friends, and crushing a major goal.

Our minds are being tricked into generating a surge of exhilaration from a very short-lived and empty source, so we continue to chase a high that will never be satisfied. We have become a slave to our technology, allowing it to control our emotional state, all the while numbing us to the real world that is happening outside of our handheld contraption.

Comparisonitis, as they call it, has become a huge epidemic, due to the rise of social media. The minute we open our apps, we are subjected to everyone's "perfect lives," commonly referred to as "highlight reels." We tune in to watch Rick, who closed on his new Malibu mansion last week; the month vacation Jim and Sally took in Europe, eating baguettes without gaining a pound; and the perfectly curated wardrobe that makes Cindy look like she fell off the cover of last month's *Vogue.* Then we go back to our own dull, mundane lives feeling more discouraged than ever.

Well, I have news for you: what you are seeing is not the entire picture. Don't forget you are only witnessing an extremely small fraction of another person's life. Until we trade our voyeurism for real-life experiences, we will be forever caught in the comparison web. So, go get some dopamine highs from that cliff dive you've been wanting to do, because that's as real as it gets, folks!

Technology from our smartphones doesn't end at social media; it also supports our incessant use of the

Internet and text messaging. It leads to other poor habits like procrastination to escape the stressors in our lives, which is ironic, since it is a surefire way to pack on even more stress. The root of procrastination is fear, to protect us from the pain associated with that fear. The fear we are experiencing is often the anticipation of a negative outcome, and not the perceived negative outcome, itself. Once we realize this, it becomes much easier to kick, knowing that the only thing to fear is fear itself. Boom. Mic drop.

Multitasking is another booster of stress and killer of productivity. The more tasks we are doing at one time, the less quality and efficiency we can dedicate to those tasks. Studies have also shown that multitasking increases production of cortisol, the hormone that causes the stress. Yup, the one that gives us that stubborn belly fat. So, all those early mornings in the gym mean squat when you're constantly diverting your focus on a million and one things.

Engaging in multitasking also results in mental fatigue. No shocker there. I mean, how productive can one really be when we are checking our texts and email every fifteen minutes? I have to keep it real with you all—no words on these pages were possible without the silencing of notifications. This book should really have a separate dedication to the all-enchanted airplane mode. You the real MVP.

There are a few other bad habits we engage in that we may not be as attuned to. One of these is the famous overcommitting. The "Yes" (Wo)Man. Is that you? Do you go to the ends of the earth to please anyone and everyone? We say "yes" for many reasons: fear of letting others down; wanting to be a team player; perceived obligation; fear of rejection; proving something to ourselves; being polite. Well, stop it. Right now. While you may think it's winning you a popularity test, it's actually sending a handwritten invitation in beautiful calligraphy to everyone who is ready to take advantage of you. It's robbing you of your precious time that could be spent dedicated to tasks that drive *your* life forward and fulfill *your* wants and needs.

Helping out is one thing, but being a doormat for anyone who is willing to walk all over you is another. There is so much power in saying "no." And the best part? Over time, people will learn to respect you for it. Now, that's a win-win. Not to mention, when we spread ourselves too thin, the outcome lacks quality, and let's be real—no one likes a half-asser.

Negative self-talk is another bad habit that seems to go completely unnoticed by most. Even when we catch ourselves, we often believe this thinking and speaking holds little weight.

Wrong. This is one of the things—if not *the* most important thing—that needs to go, if we want to achieve great success and live a happy life.

Words have a profound influence on our perception of reality. Most of us would never dream of speaking to others the way we speak to ourselves. This is another area where energy comes into play: words carry a ton of it. They are the difference between eliciting a positive outlook on our day versus a negative one. Just think of what that can do to our moods over time.

Worrying, self-criticism, and playing the victim are just a few ways in which we corner ourselves into negative self-talk. Take the time to consciously listen to how you speak to and about yourself, then practice shifting your language from words of pain to power. The less we subject ourselves to this type of self-inflicted abuse, the closer we come to gratitude for all of the awesomeness we possess to design a kick-ass life.

I probably don't have to tell you that complaining fosters a negative attitude. Focusing on the negative always brings in more negative because it's all you see and all you will remember. And, like the old saying goes, "misery loves company." Focusing on what is going wrong sinks you deeper into your pity party and results in less action to change your current situation.

It is important to realize that there will always be a reason to complain if we look for one. Adopting the attitude that adversity is an opportunity to learn and grow is completely life-changing. Hindsight often shows us that when something is removed from our life, something better takes its place.

One major bad habit I catch my clients really giving a run for its money is self-sabotage. It took me awhile to recognize when I was in my own self-sabotaging mode.

I mentioned my tendency to binge years ago. I had this unrealistic expectation of what my body composition should be at all times, so, whenever I fell short, I threw the baby out with the bathwater and the food-eating contest commenced. (Although it was only me I was competing with... You can imagine how that went.) This is like getting a flat tire and going ahead and slashing the other three. We are human, and life is not linear. We will have ups and downs, but when we learn how to pick ourselves up and dust ourselves off after each fall, we get closer and closer to our goals over time.

A final habit I believe is critical to bring attention to is our tendency to fall prey to our limiting beliefs. We all have them, and they're a prime reason we hold ourselves back in life. They are often created by what external sources have taught us: family, friends, media, education, etc. Many of us are raised in a household or culture where we were taught to go to school, get a college degree, work at a 9-5, get married, have children, save for retirement, retire at sixty-two… then die. Morbid, yes. But this is nothing you haven't been exposed to, yourselves. We go into autopilot, operating in the box that was created for us, unconsciously going through the motions without ever questioning these beliefs. And, as a result, greatly limiting our potential.

Why do we hold so tightly to these beliefs when it can seem so obvious how unhealthy they may be? *Cognitive dissonance* is a concept that supports such behavior. In a nutshell, when one is presented with evidence that works against a person's core beliefs, the new evidence cannot be accepted. Since it is very important to protect the core belief, we tend to rationalize, ignore, and even deny anything that doesn't align with that belief to avoid discomfort. You can see how deep-seated this particular habit can be and how crucial it is to dig in and release it. This just goes to show you we are the only ones in our way.

At the end of the day, our habits become our routine and our routine eventually becomes the life we're living today. If we're currently in a situation that doesn't make us happy, it is likely we can trace it back to the little things we're doing every day. The behaviors we engage in on a daily basis slowly carve out our life's path, sending a to-do list to the Universe to send us whatever it is we need along the ride.

So, let go of those pesky habits that weigh you down, and tell the Universe you're ready to bring in some epic shit!

CHAPTER 8:

What Got You Here Won't Get You There

By NOW, IT'S PROBABLY clear that clutter-free is the way to be. An organized and simplified existence helps us to create clarity and mental focus, as well as reduce stress. But, above all, it opens our eyes to who we are at our core, so we can stop answering to others and instead answer to our hearts.

When it all comes down to our time on Earth, it is not about ownership or status. The purpose of every action we take or choice we make is to elicit a feeling. Once we discover this, our draw to accumulate things and people and habits that don't align with who we are no longer matters. We think from the end of how we want to *feel* and that becomes our focus. We may think we want a Ferrari, but maybe we just want the feeling of freedom with the wind in our hair or, perhaps, the attention we were always starved of. Maybe we just want love and acceptance, to fill a void we've been missing.

Living a life of less is about finding ourselves underneath all of the distractions. Something incredible happens when you're no longer weighed down by the unimportant things. So much can be revealed when we are unblocked, unchained, light, and free. Letting go of everything we've built an attachment to, including the expectations of others about who we should be, is one of the most significant things we can do while we're alive.

But it will not be easy. It's going to take a lot of dedication and energy to un-become who we thought ourselves to be for all these years, so we can become who we are today. It's not going to be easy to escape the traps set all around us that try to lure us back to our old lives.

Nothing changes if nothing changes. We must draw a line in the sand, declaring from this day forward we are not willing to live like we have been anymore.

It is time to let go of everything that has ever held you back:

- ✓ Your junk.
- ✓ Your toxic relationships.
- ✓ Your unserving habits.
- ✓ Your old stories.
- ✓ Your false identity.
- ✓ Your past.
- ✓ Your excuses.
- ✓ Your fear.

You are ready to live a life full of intention because you now know who you are and what it is you genuinely want. Your mission becomes easier, your purpose clearer. The steps you need to put into action to design your new life happen with ease. You are now living a life of meaning, because you have made the conscious decision to prioritize what is truly important.

Please remember: *you* are in control of your destiny. You deserve the best life, and you have all the power in the world to create an existence full of pure joy and happiness.

It all just starts with letting go.

How to Apply The Less Effect to Your Life

The Less Effect is an online course for anyone feeling overwhelmed and unfulfilled who is looking to uncover their true passion to create a life of joy and meaning. It is also for successful entrepreneurs who want to remove subconscious limitations, allowing you to get to the next level in your business.

So many of us spend a large part of our lives living in an old, unserving story that blocks us from our true potential. Through this framework, you will unlock the power to rewrite your story by removing attachments holding you back and uncover your core identity to design the life you've always dreamed of.

Each phase of the course is dedicated to one of three key life areas:

* Physical environment
* Social environment
* Habitual environment

The course outlines the steps to identifying aspects of our environment that are hindering us and then how to carefully remove them from our lives. This is complemented by exercises that focus on becoming more intentional in attracting surroundings that align with our true identity. Each module builds on each other to develop your level of confidence in following your passion to design your most meaningful life.

One Client's Experience: Alex Gonzalez

Opportunity. Honesty. Integrity.

These are words that often get thrown around in our everyday lives. We may say things like, "I had the opportunity to meet someone interesting today," or, "What a great opportunity," when speaking of someone or even ourselves, when new job placement is involved or if we are able to catch a great show or speaker.

Often we use honesty and integrity to help us gauge those around us and give us a scale for how we see others. But how often do we give ourselves "opportunity"? How often are we truly "honest" with ourselves, hold ourselves to a standard of "integrity," and truly look at ourselves, to get to know who we really are?

Enter *The Less Effect.*

The Less Effect allowed me to really get out of my comfort zone and look at my life as if I was a third person, and get to know the most important person in my life... me. It forced me to give myself the opportunity to carve out time... real time, to get to know how I function, what things make me comfortable, what I need in my life, and, more importantly, what I don't need. It was a way to be truly honest with myself about my living space, my social and family circles, the people I allowed in my life, my struggles, my anxieties, what makes me truly happy, and what doesn't.

It was a way to hold my self accountable for the hierarchy of value I gave to the situations and experiences I've allowed myself or kept coming back to, the "stuff" I kept, and all of the things that encompass what one would consider to be the environment of your life—the space where I lived not only physically but in my heart and mind, as well.

Throughout my experience with *The Less Effect,* I found myself getting rid of so much dead weight that had held me down from being the best version of myself. I was able to get to a point in my life environment that didn't feel so bogged down and overwhelming, and everyday tasks became so much easier.

My workflow and productivity was immensely heightened, and I was able to instantly get to projects with ease. I no longer had to expend the energy to deal with the clutter of my environment and focus that energy on the productivity of my day. The "Stuff" I kept around—papers, boxes of junk, magazines, books, clothing (ugh... the clothing)—that I was able to sell or donate and then take back my physical space, which gave me a clearer headspace.

You would be surprised how much space you actually have when it is not holding the things you never touch and are really only there to gather dust. Things that we sometimes hold onto because it's our "Stuff" that we may feel gives us some sense of meaning or some sense of validation. Even those things we may give sentimental value towards that, if you're honest with yourself, we really don't need. It felt so good to give to those who needed it more. I learned that giving is really its own gift.

One of the aspects that really shook the ground for me was taking a real look at my social circle. The people who were in my life (including family), who created an effect of positivity or negativity, to truly ask if those people still belonged in my every day. If I should limit my exposure and allow myself to truly blossom, or if I needed more of the positivity I was getting and perhaps befriend more people who inspired and generated such an effect. Learning to say "no" sometimes. Not to mention learning to ask myself the question, "What value do I myself give to this relationship?" Holding your own self accountable and truly challenging yourself to be at the level of those you admire. No need to reinvent the wheel, if you know someone who is doing it right. Your own wheel will follow.

To bring it all together, *The Less Effect* is a real way to give you perspective. Your life is your own. Take hold and give it purpose. It gave me a way to see paths to goals I've had and to see newer and better goals to strive for. Life is something that will knock you down, so put on some damn gloves, and jump in that ring! Time is our most precious commodity and how and with whom we use it is the value you give to yourself.

Allow *The Less Effect* to streamline your life and accomplish things that, in the past, may have seemed daunting that now can be easily attainable goals.

The Less Effect was a gift to me, and Samantha Joy is a gift to the world. Her resilience and the sheer power of her will has transformed these ideas into something to behold that will take your life and rock it to the core. It will shake things up in such a good way, you will never want to live your life as you once had.

"And once you're awake, you shall remain awake eternally."

—Nietzsche

The Less Effect has allowed me to carve a path that will take me across the country to follow a career path that, before, I could only dream about. Give yourself this gift. Who you are today and who you will be is entirely up to you, and *The Less Effect* will help you get there.

***

To receive updates on enrollment for the next course opening, please email:

hello@thelesseffect.com

ACKNOWLEDGMENTS

*I*F YOU'VE GOTTEN THIS FAR in the book, I want to thank you. Thank you for reading this message that I could not be more passionate about, and thank you for becoming awake to your own life in where you may be holding yourself back. I'm so excited for what you're about to create.

I would also like to thank the following people who made this book possible:

~AJ Mihrzad, for giving me the kick in the ass I needed to finally write a book, and your endless knowledge, support, and belief through the process.

~Matt & Caleb Maddix, for, no matter how busy these two are saving the world, always making time for a friend with dreams.

~My mother, Deborah, for teaching me her "woo-woo" ways and always believing in my abilities, no matter what crazy ideas I throw at her.

~*The Less Effect* Live Beta Focus Group, 1.0: Alex, Judy, Chase, Hiromi, Camilla, Debbie, Linda, Danielle, Amad, Juliana, and Sylvia, for investing in my baby and rocking incredible transformations!

~Kathryn, my editor, for making my first book a beautiful success.

ABOUT SAMANTHA

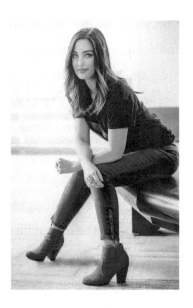

S AMANTHA JOY is a Mindset & Empowerment Coach to aspiring entrepreneurs and influencers. Her coaching approach focuses on the concept of *minimalism,* where she enables others to shift their identity to their most authentic self by decluttering aspects of their life rooted in an old story.

She spent the last year on her own personal journey, following and crafting *The Less Effect* framework, which has brought her immense happiness and purpose, as it has to many others.

Samantha grew up in the Northeast in the small suburb of Farmington, Connecticut, and she has lived in six major cities since then. Denver, Colorado, where she currently resides, is her favorite by far—no coincidence, after applying her course framework to her own life.

Samantha has a passion for writing, body movement, social impact, and entrepreneurship. Her free time is spent hiking in the mountains with her dog, Juliett, dining out at the hottest new vegan joint, fostering meaningful relationships over decaf coffee, reading personal development in the bathtub, and jetting off on a plane to her next adventure (at least once per year). Samantha believes travel and service to others are life's greatest teachers.

Samantha Joy launched her new publishing house, Landon Hail Press, in 2022 and serves as editor-in-chief for a host of wise, exciting new publications, including a line of illustrated children's books great for every family.

***

Made in United States
Troutdale, OR
03/12/2024

18405319R00072